GEE WHIZ, G-TUBE!

by Emily & Kyrie Christensen
editing & design by Nathan Christensen

HWC
PRESS

Do you see this tube in my nose?

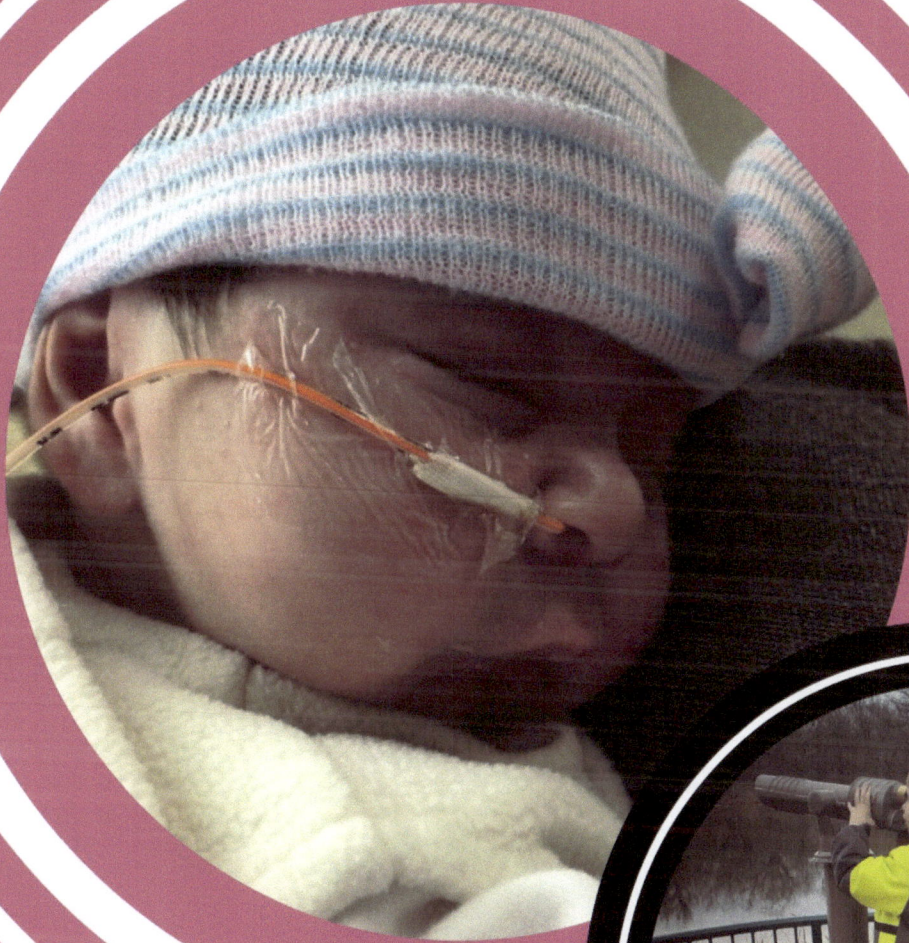
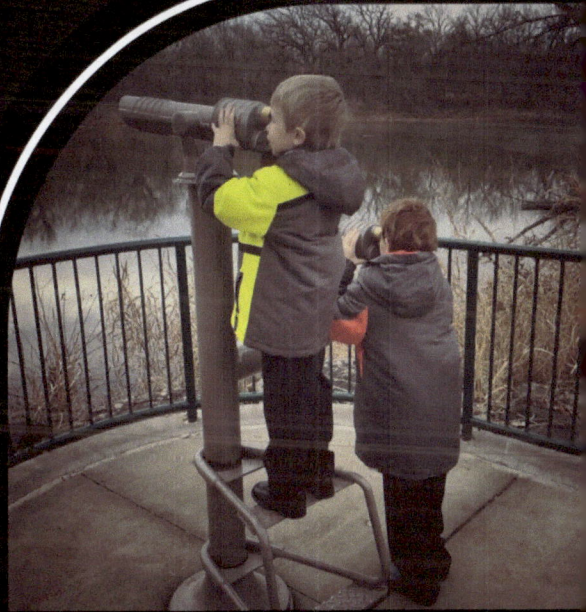

It used to
follow me
everywhere.

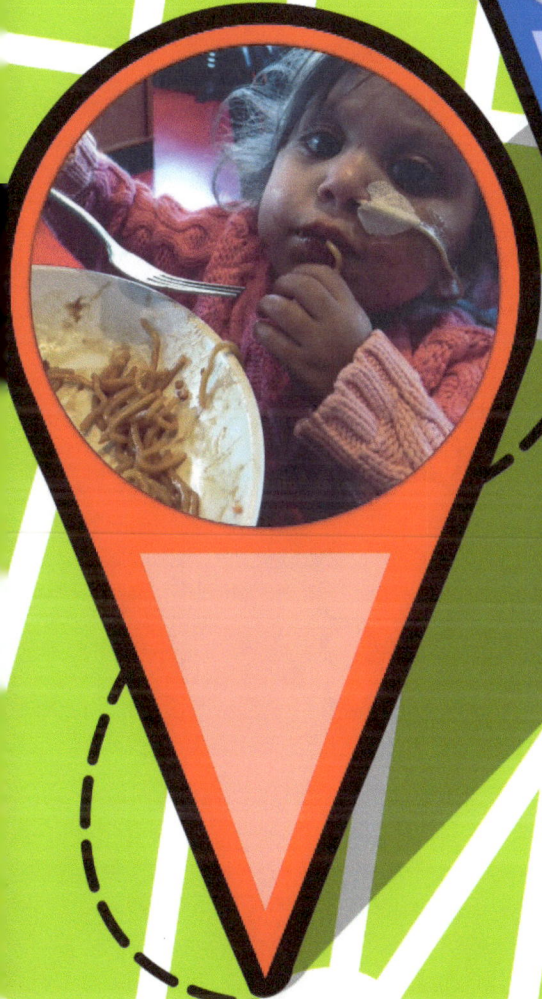

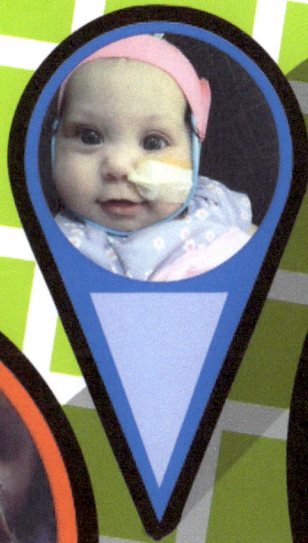

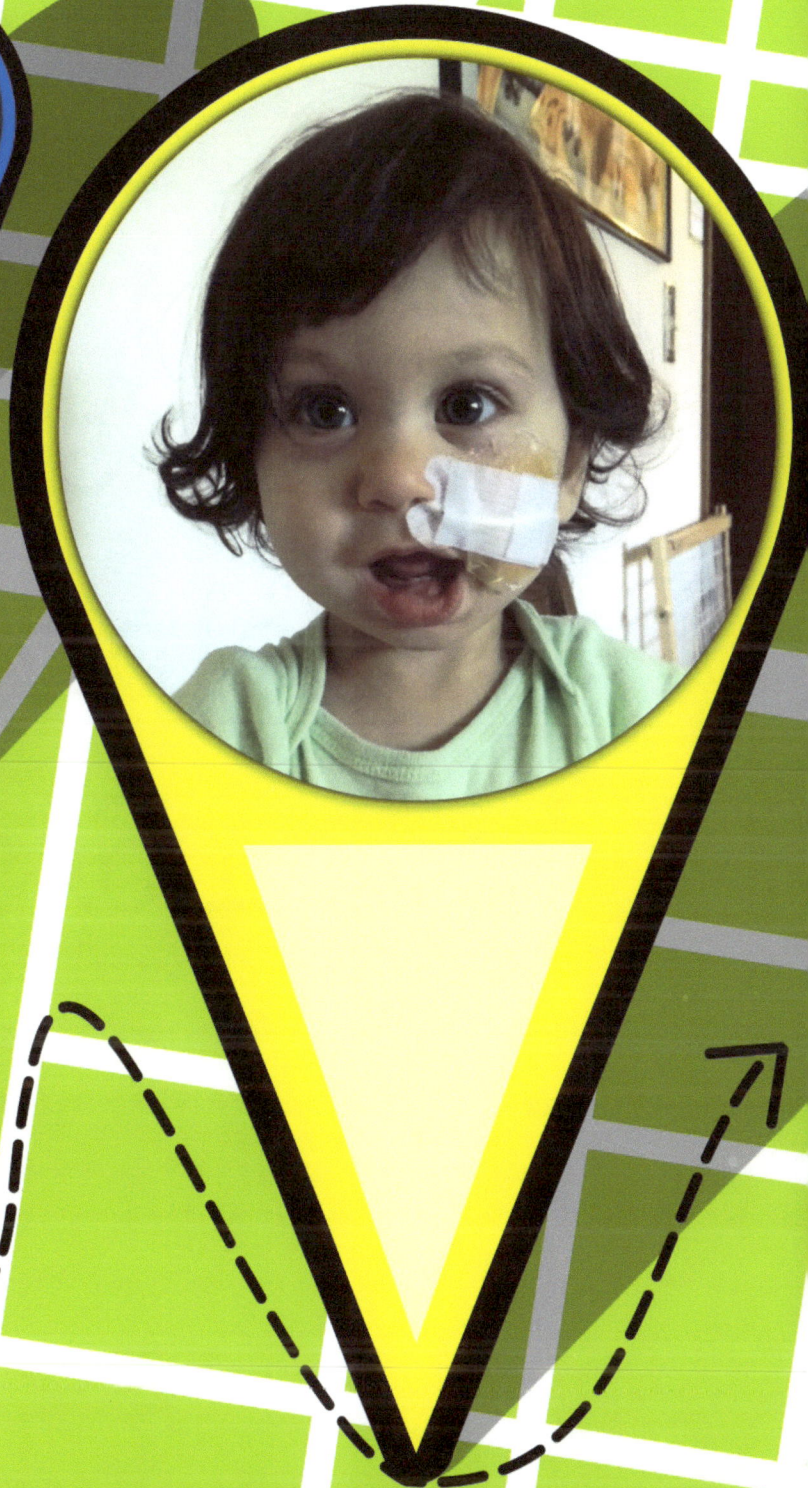

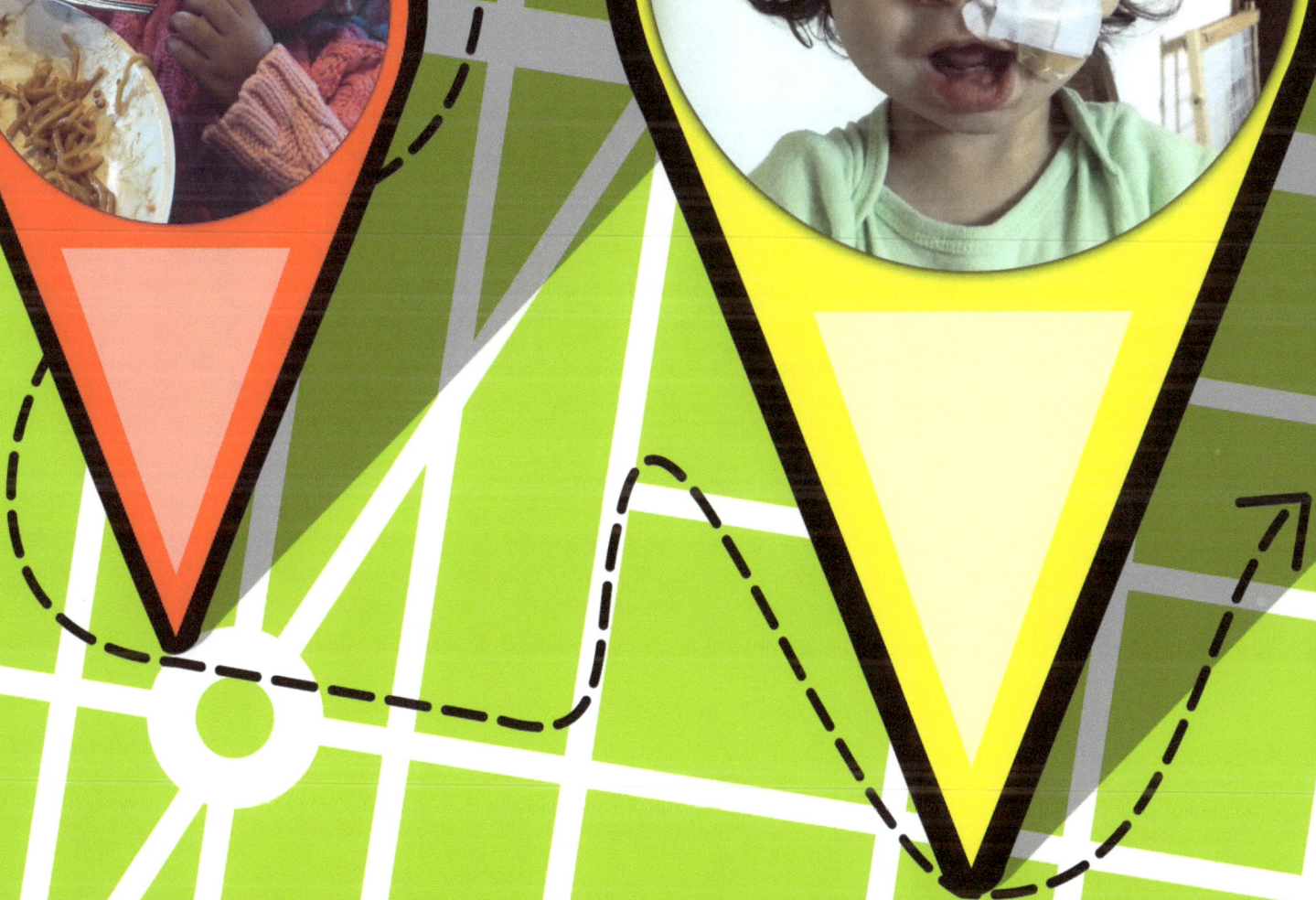

It was supposed to help me grow big and strong.

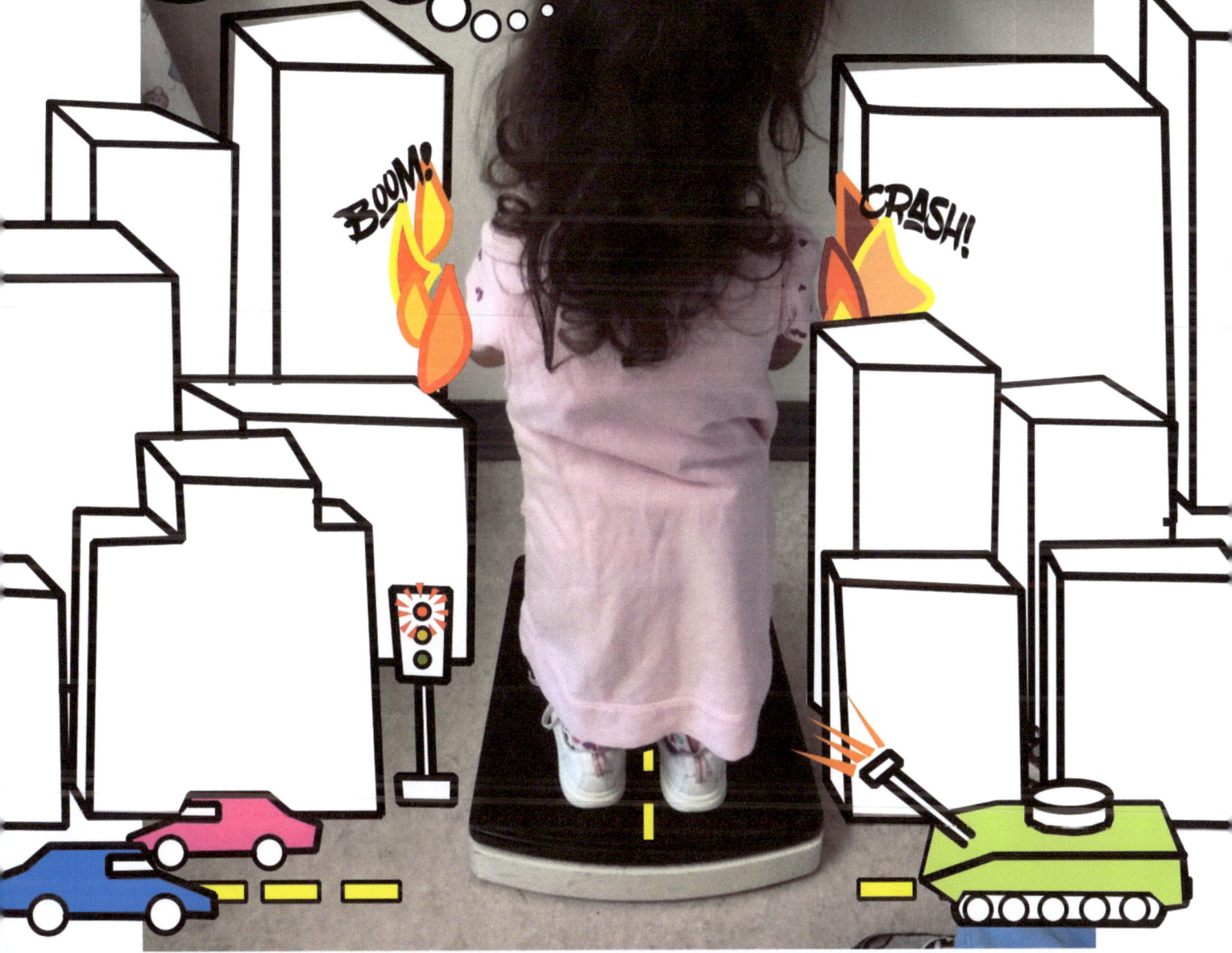

My parents tried to make it look all cute...

but they couldn't fool me.

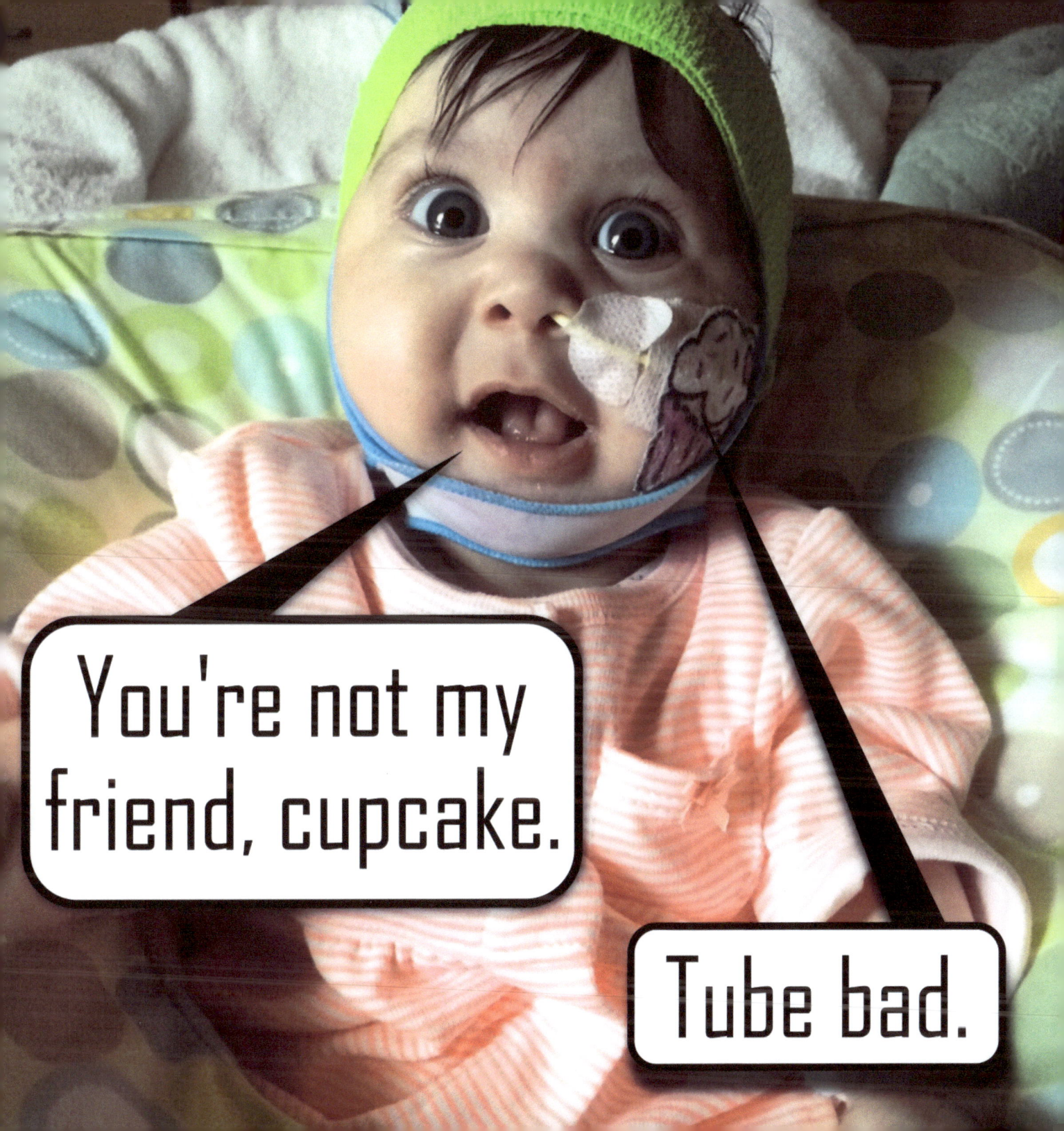

Maybe I needed it, but I sure didn't like it.

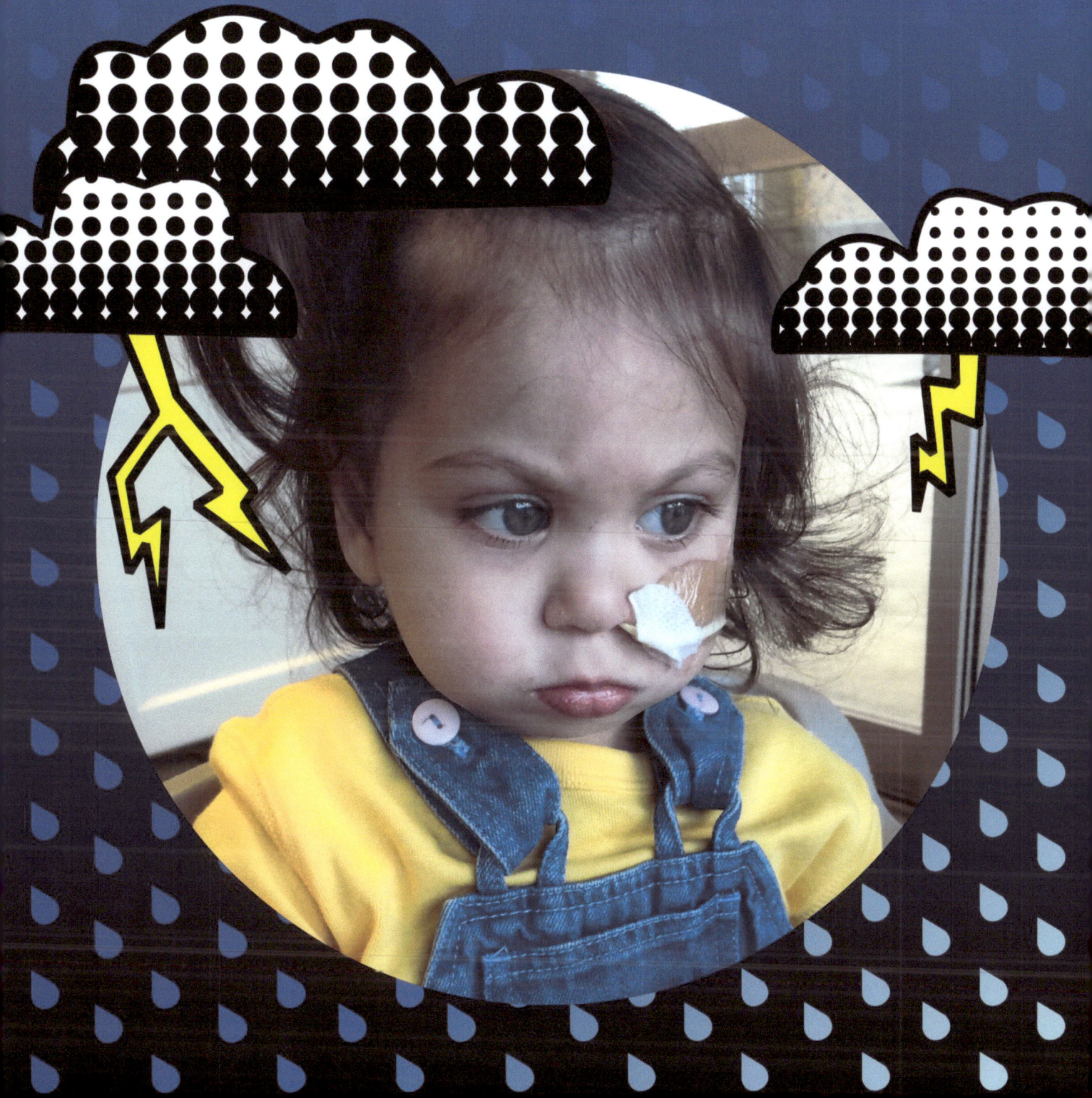

This nose just wasn't big enough for the both of us.

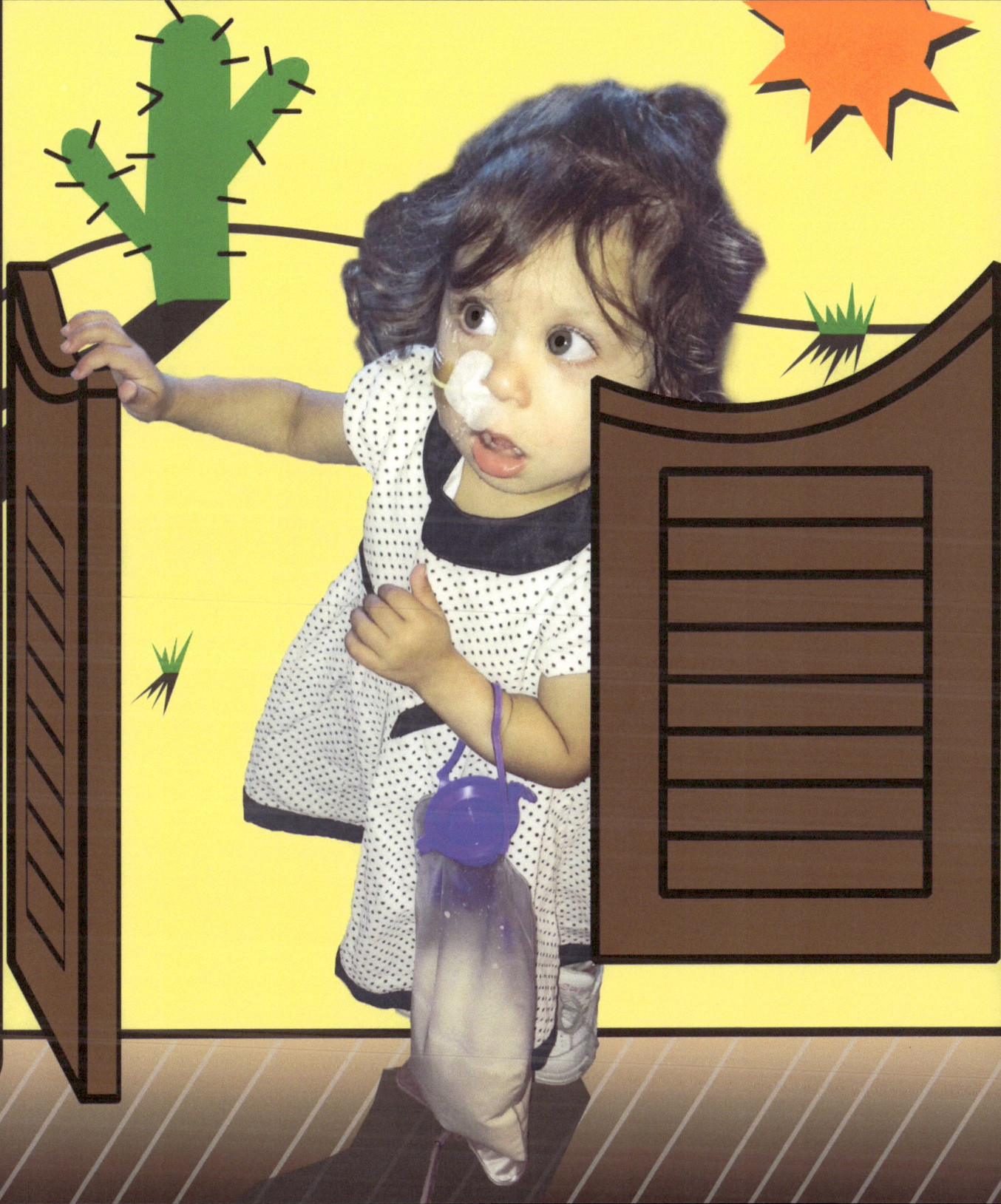

So I called my friends together.

"THE CREW"

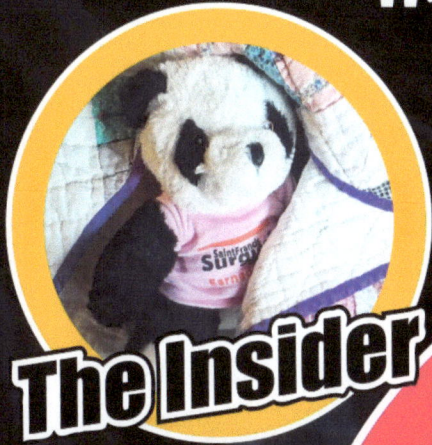

The Insider

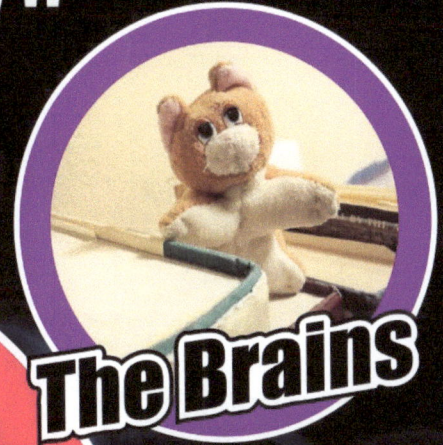

The Brains

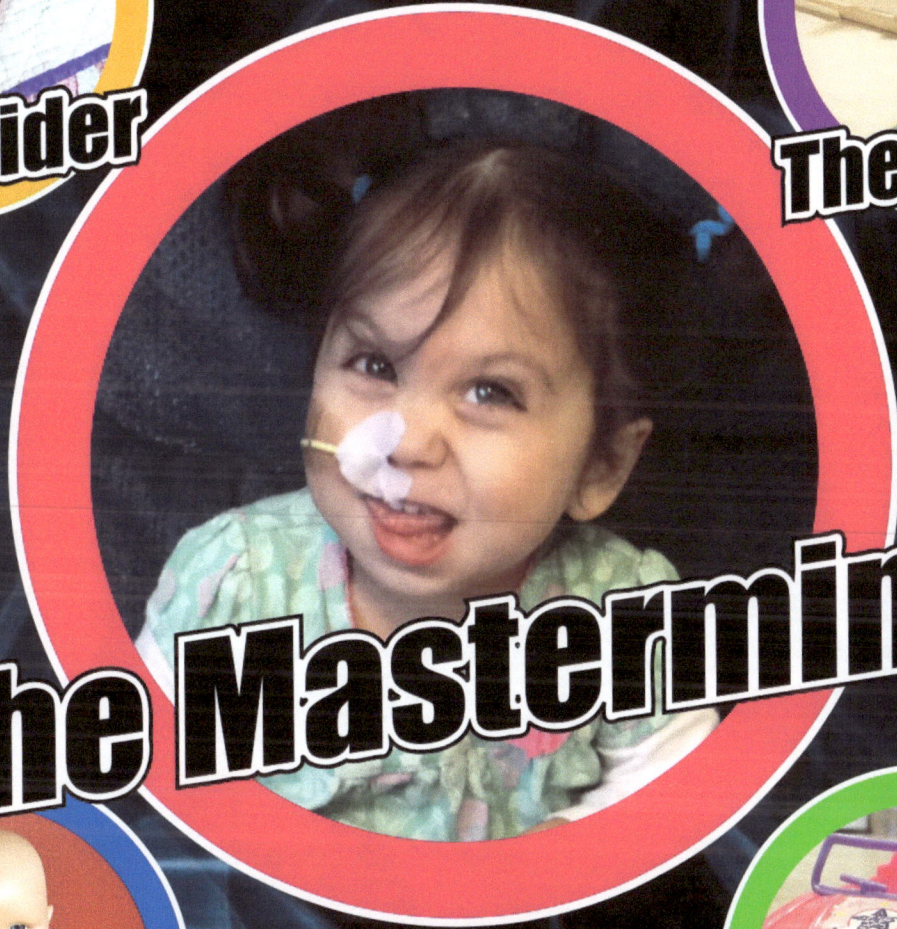

The Mastermind

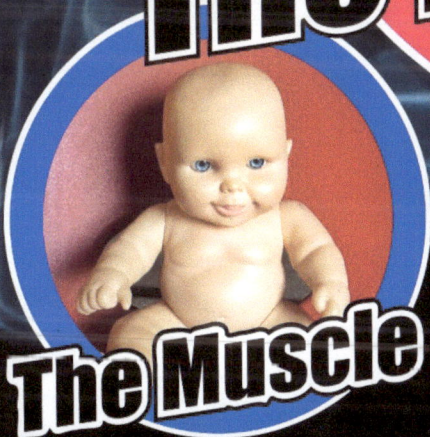

The Muscle

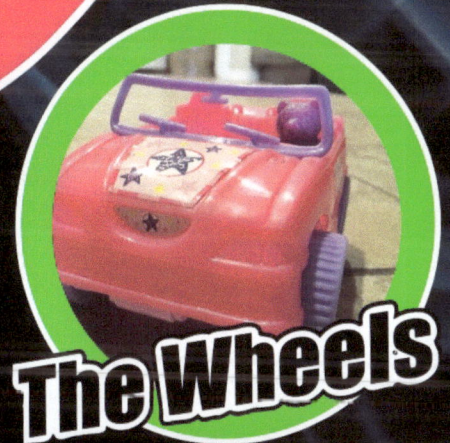

The Wheels

We came up with a daring plan.

1.

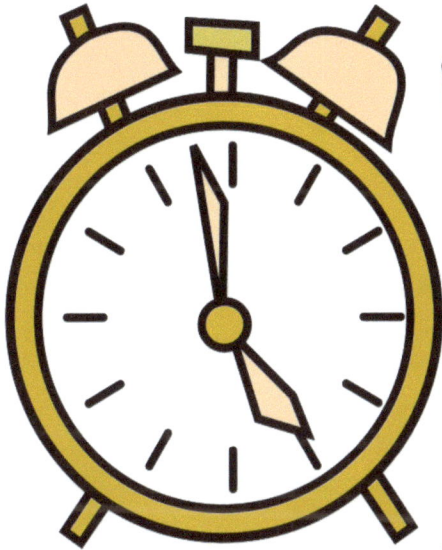

2.

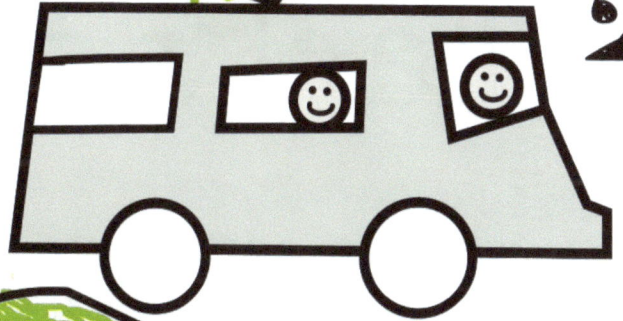

3.

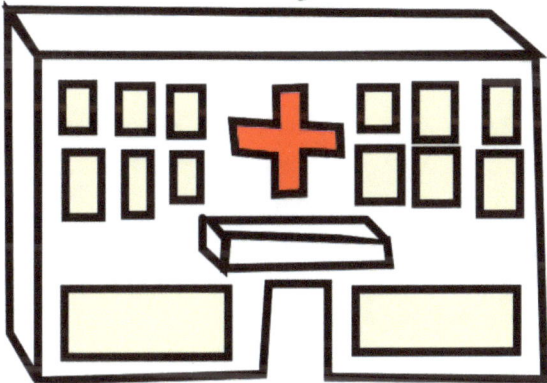

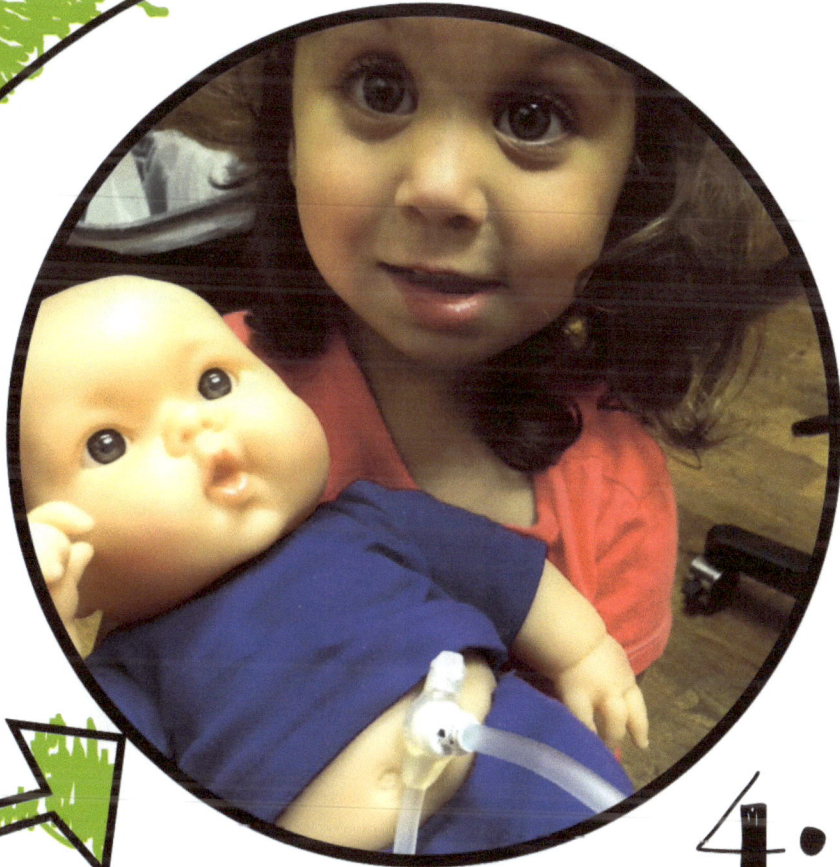

4.

Early one morning, we slipped into the hospital, and put on our disguises.

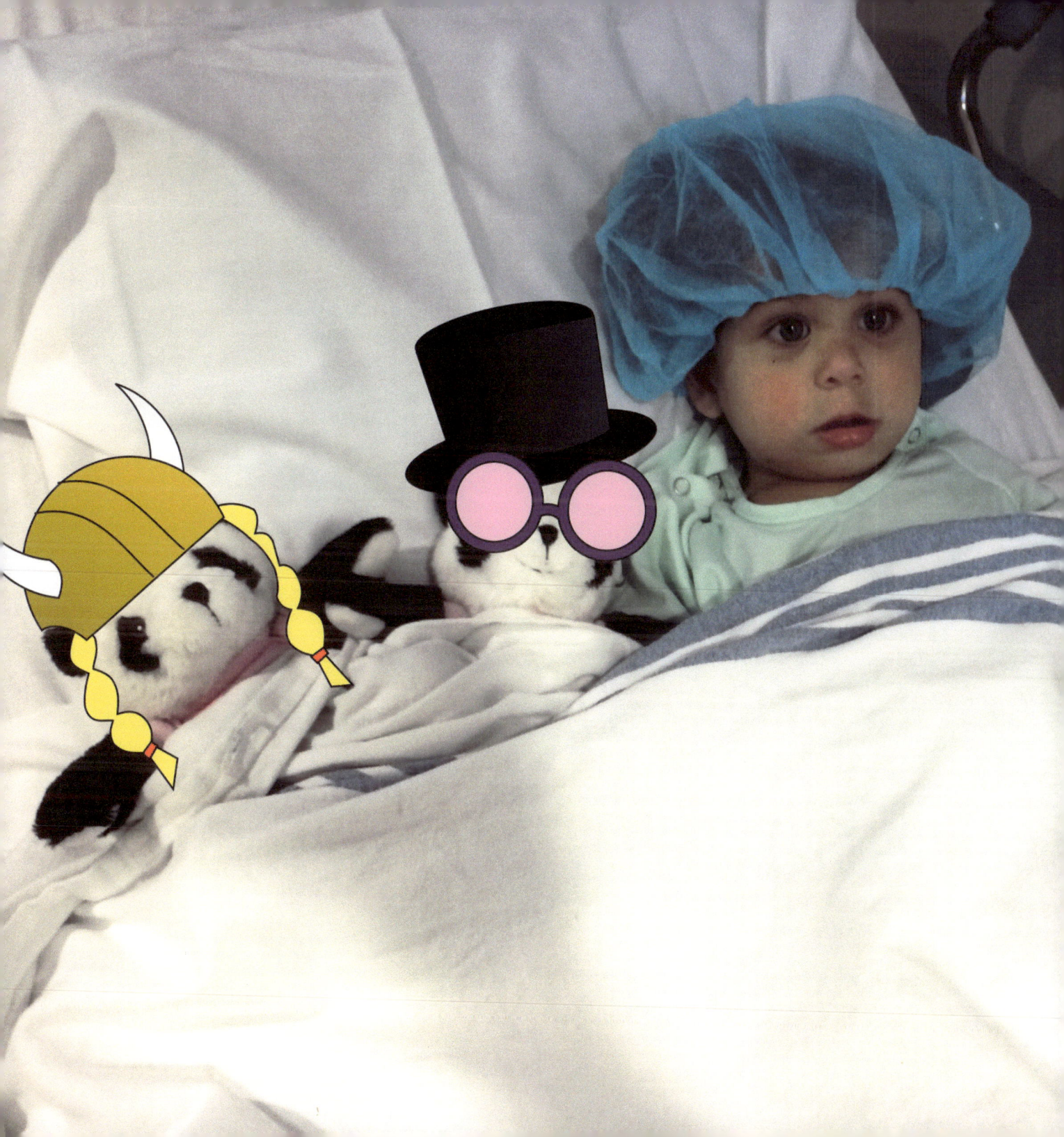

After waiting for a while, a kind doctor arrived. He gave me some medicine that made me so sleepy.

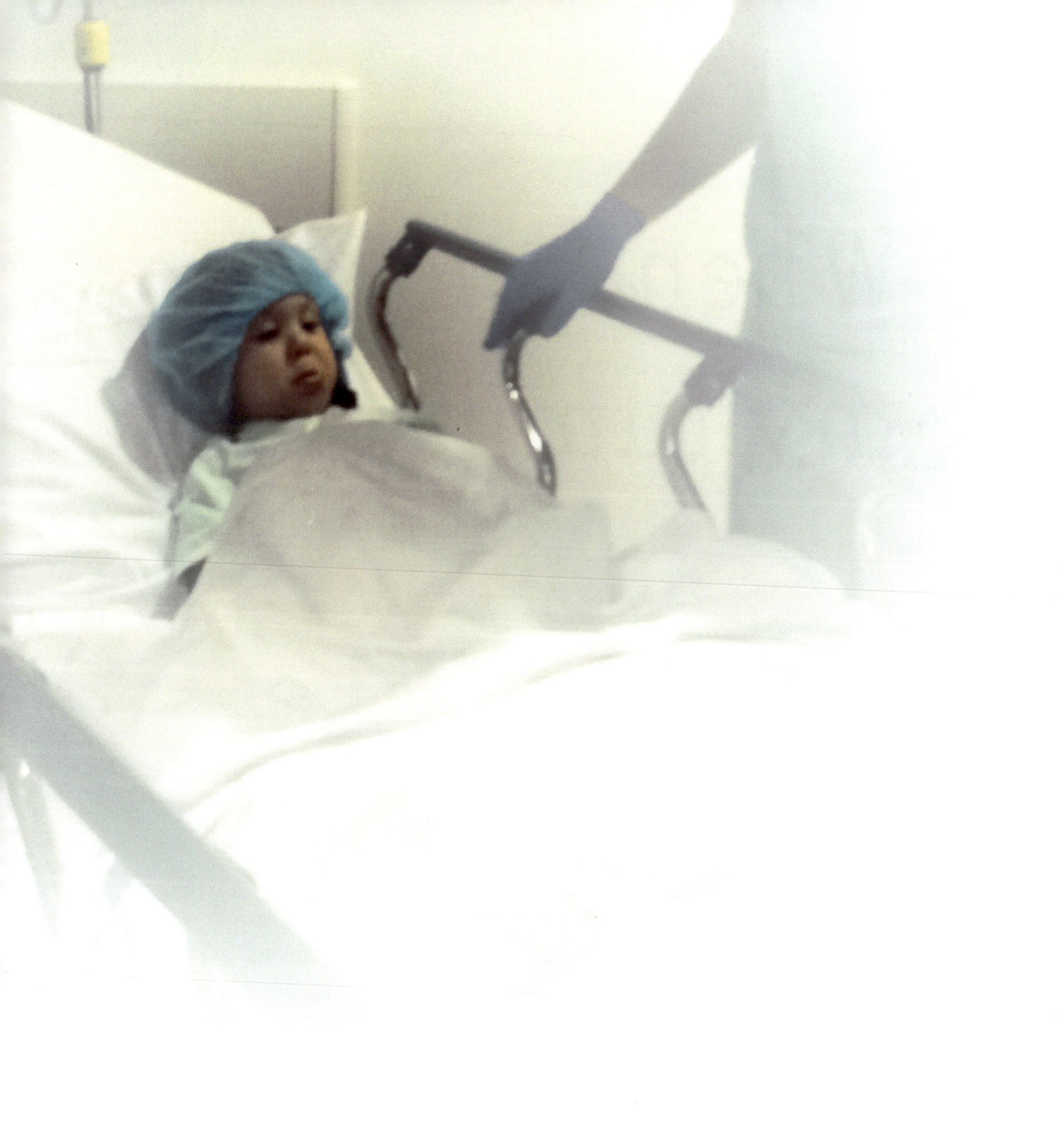

When I woke up,
my tummy hurt.

I did not like
that at all.

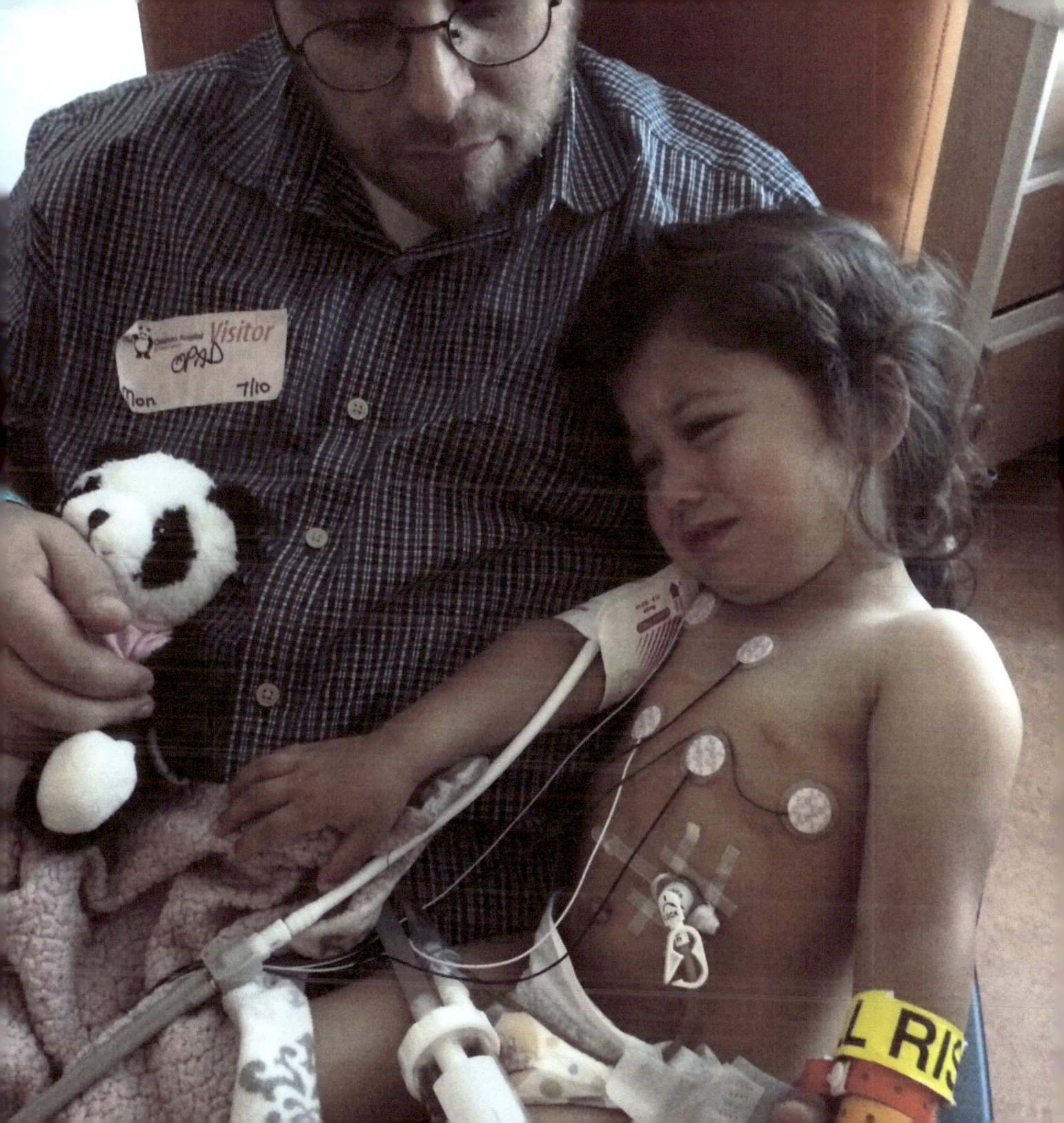

But I started feeling better the next day.

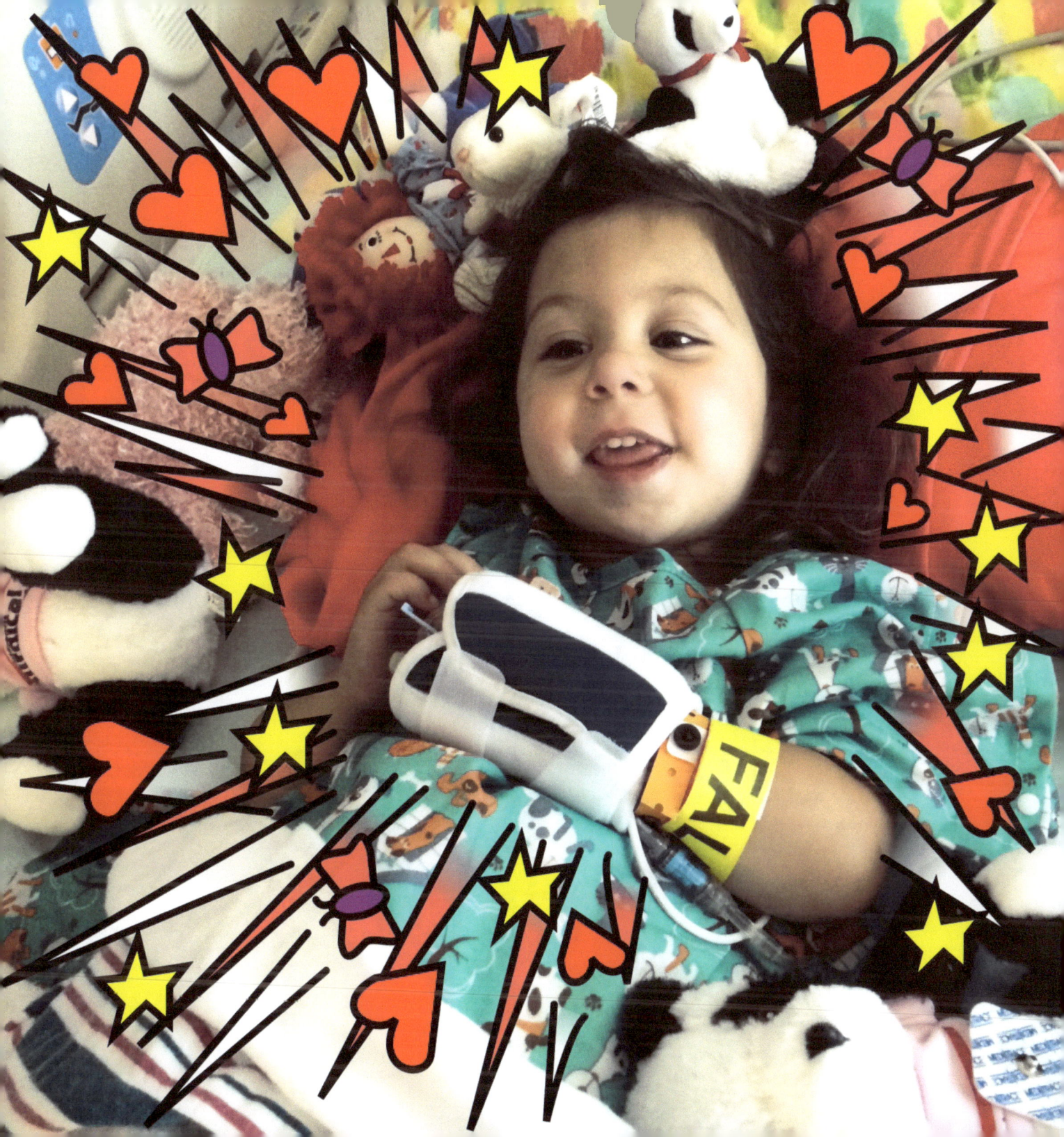

I had to stay in the hospital for so long! The doctor wanted to be sure I was ok.

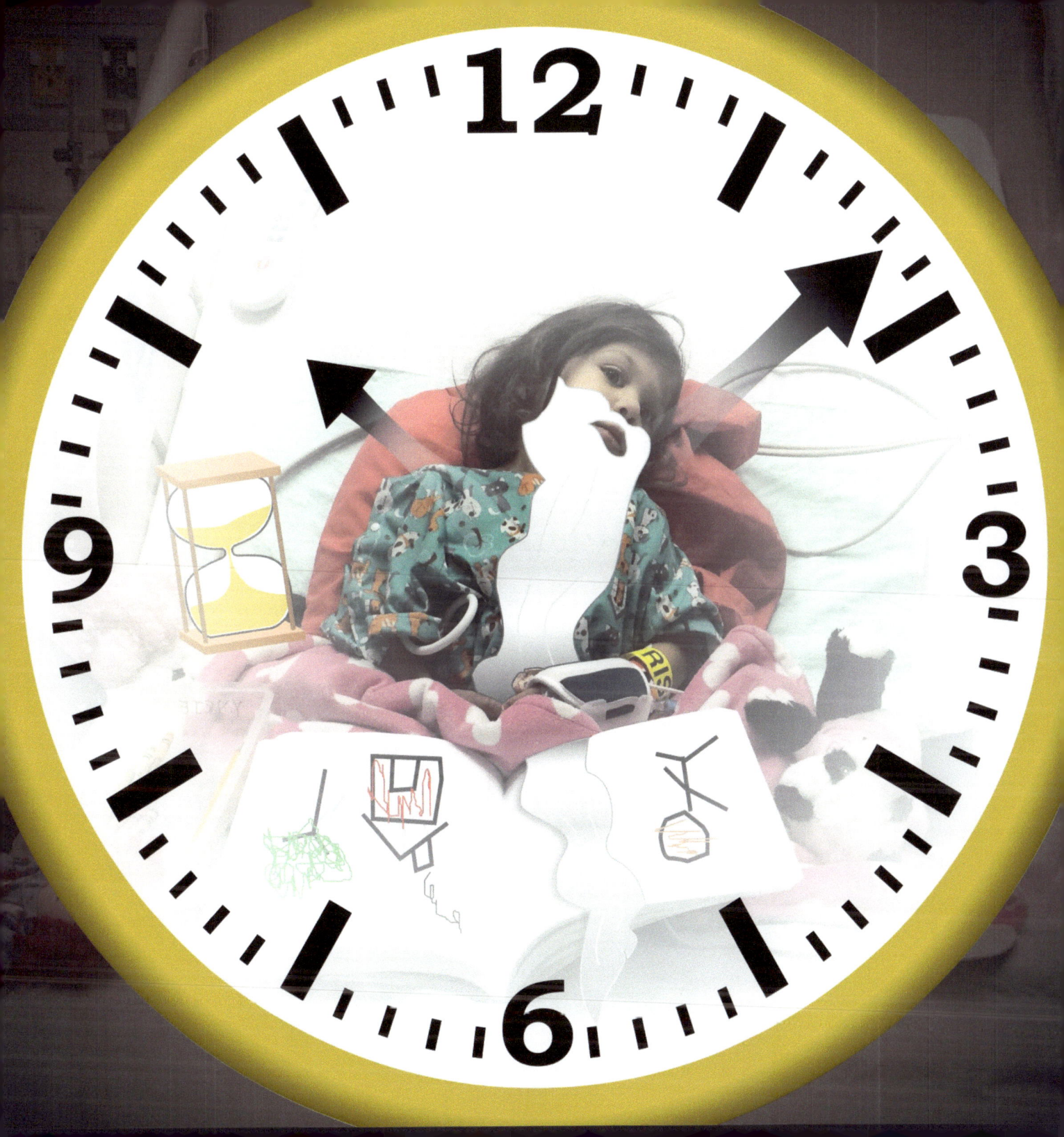

In the hospital,
I got to eat
all the slurpy
and jiggly
treats I wanted.

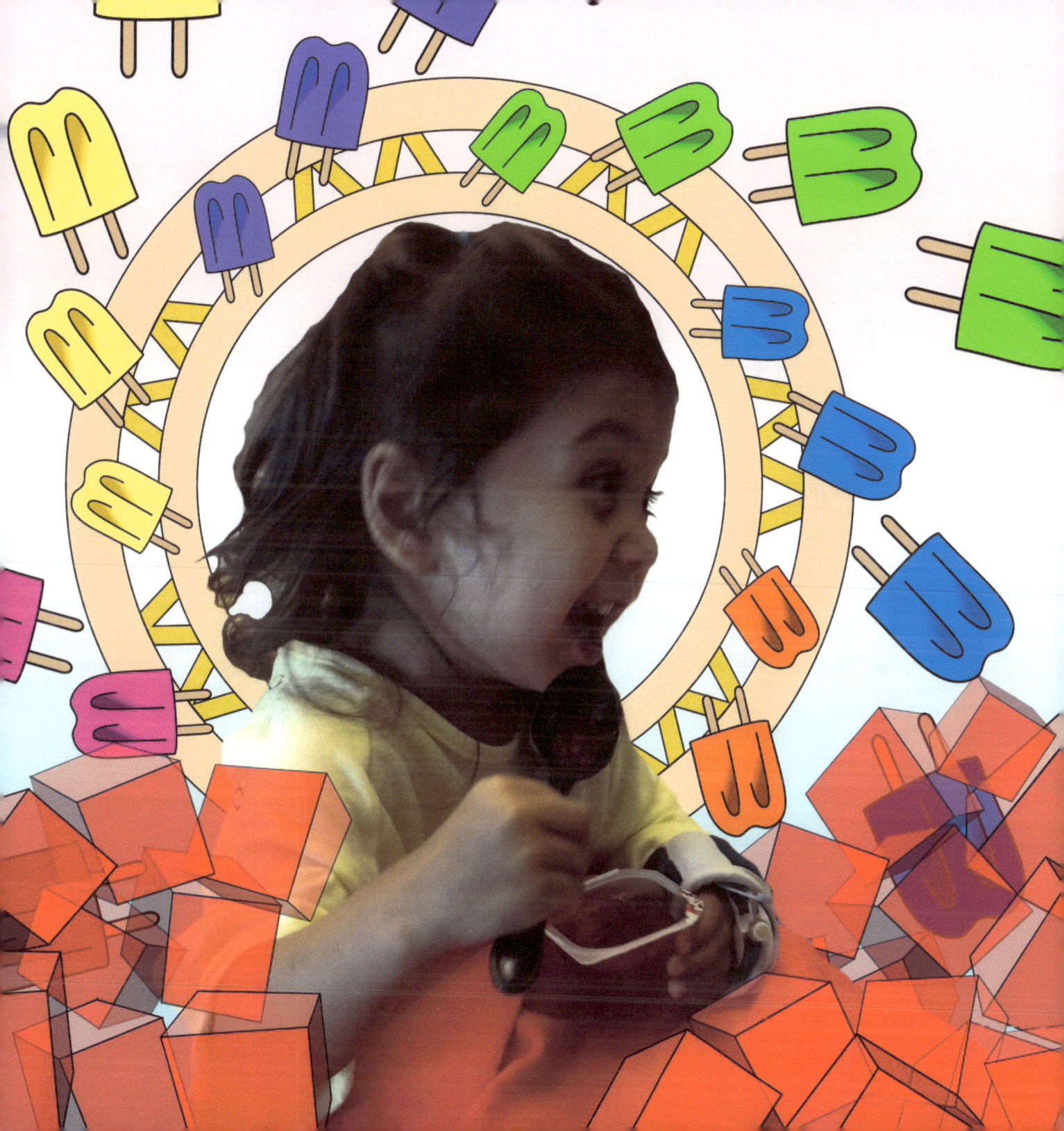

And there were
fun things
to play with.

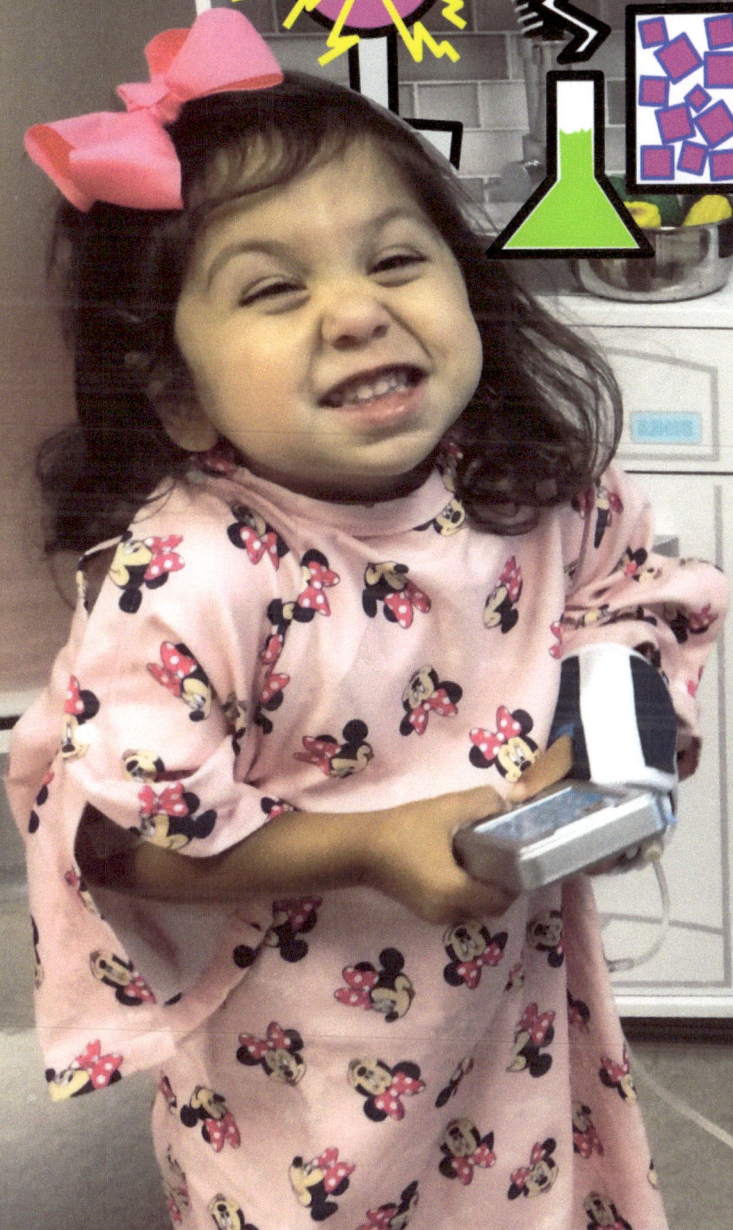
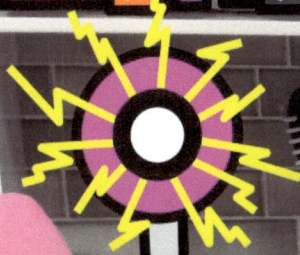
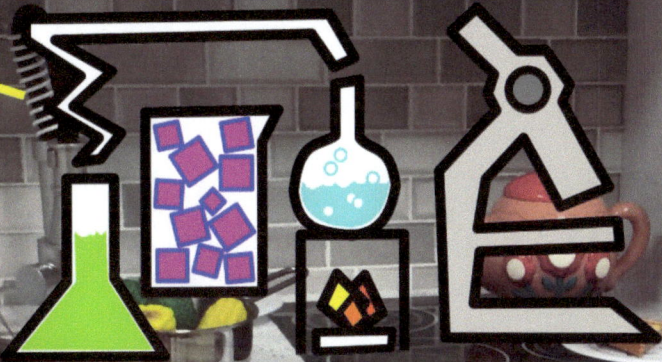
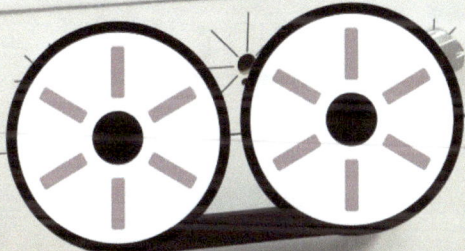
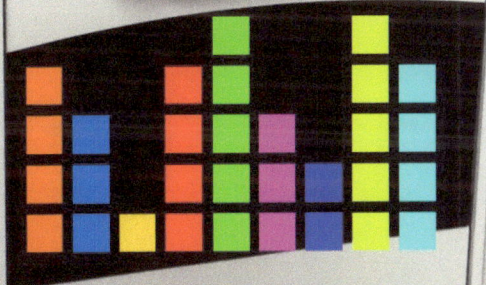
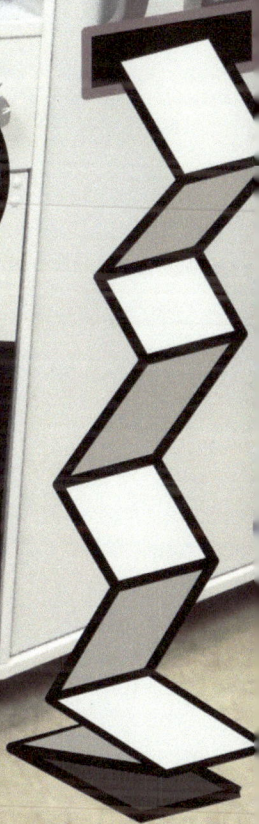

But have you discovered the very best part of it all?

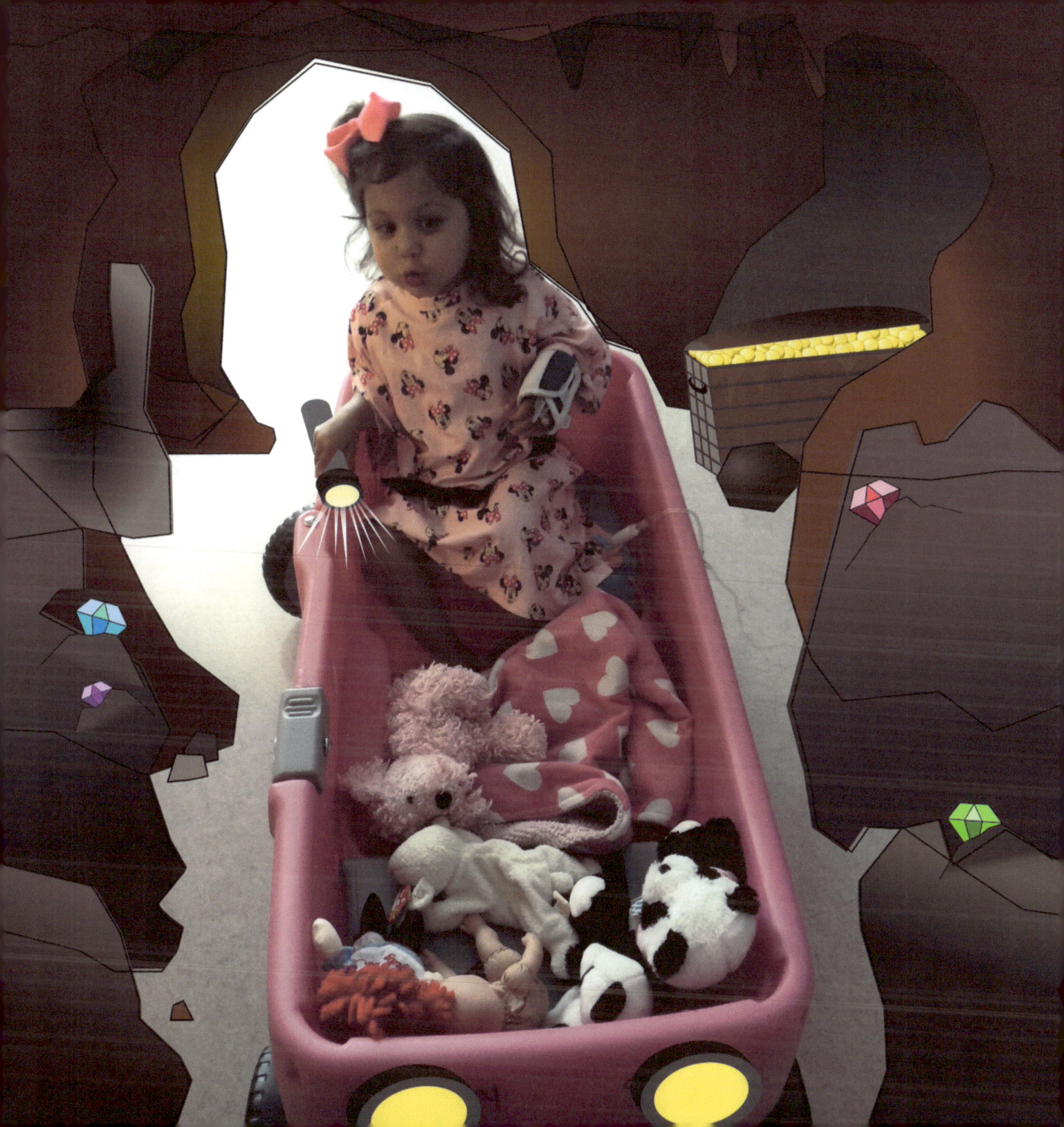

No more tube
in my nose!!!

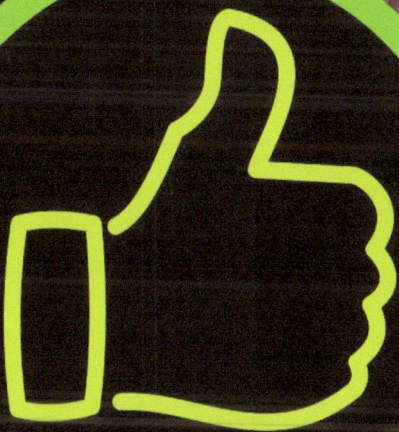

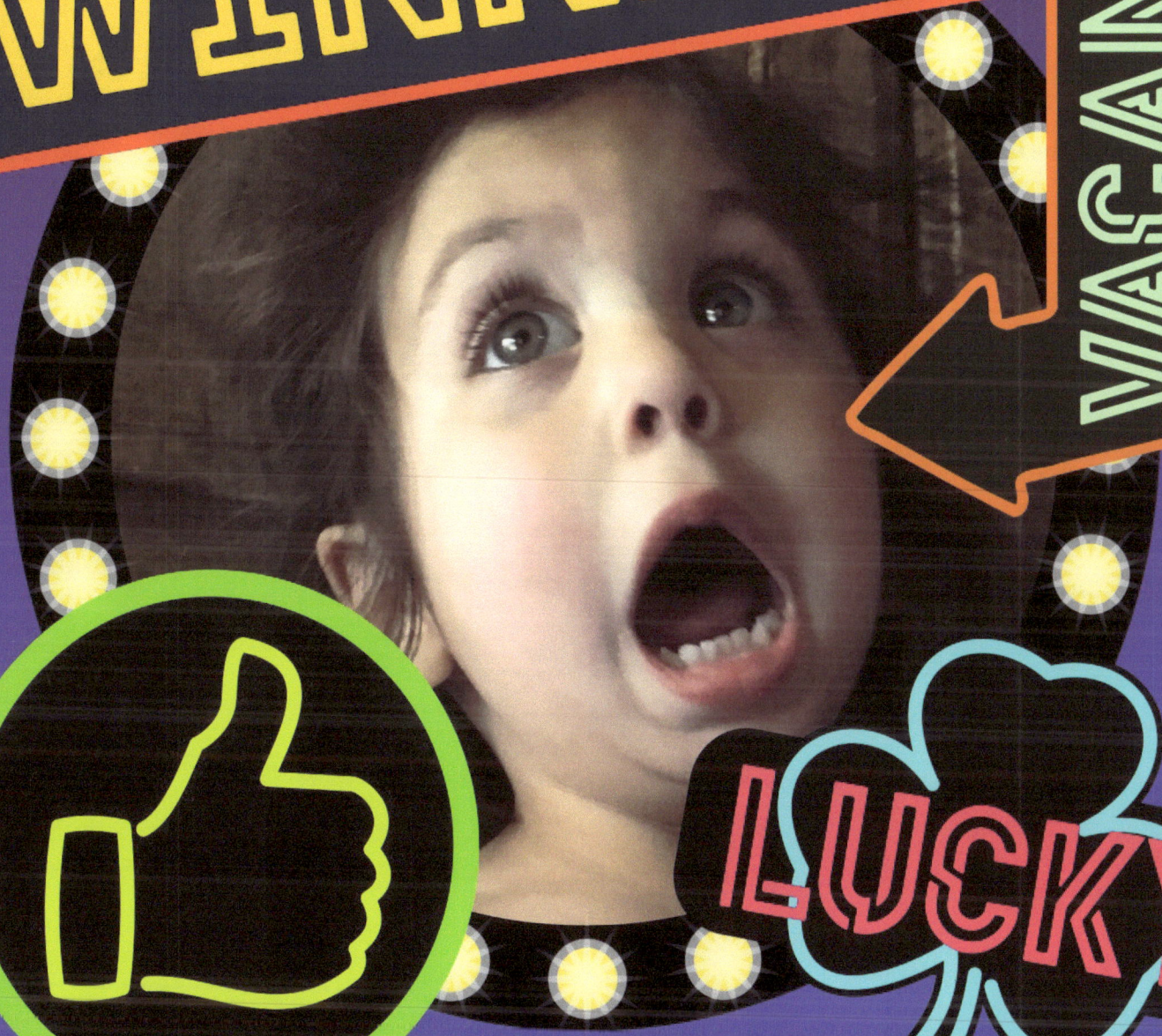

It's in my tummy, instead.

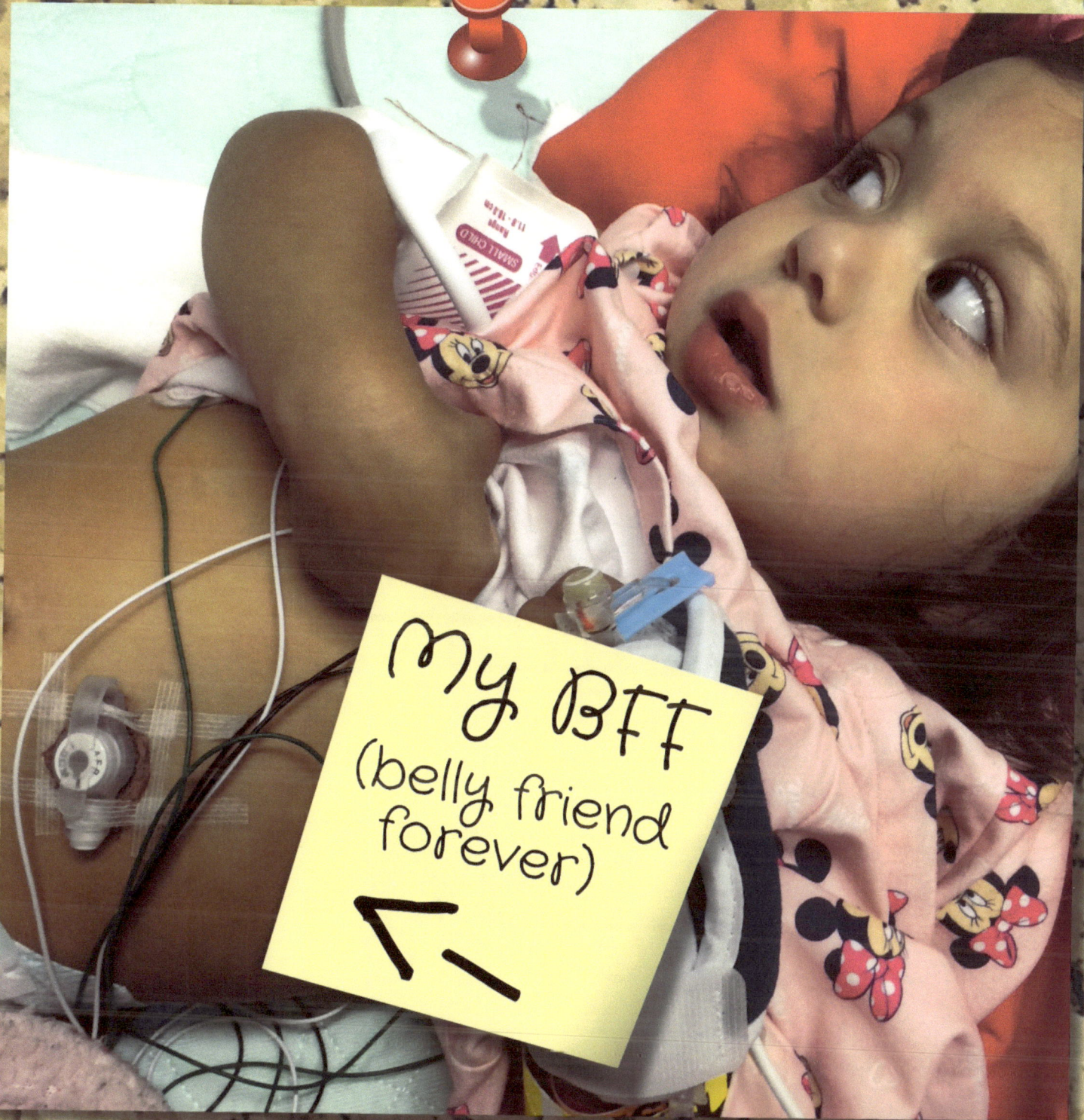

My BFF
(belly friend
forever)
←

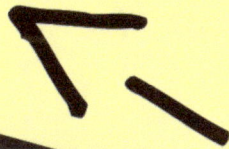

I can eat
with both
my mouth <u>and</u>
my tummy.

Can you do that?

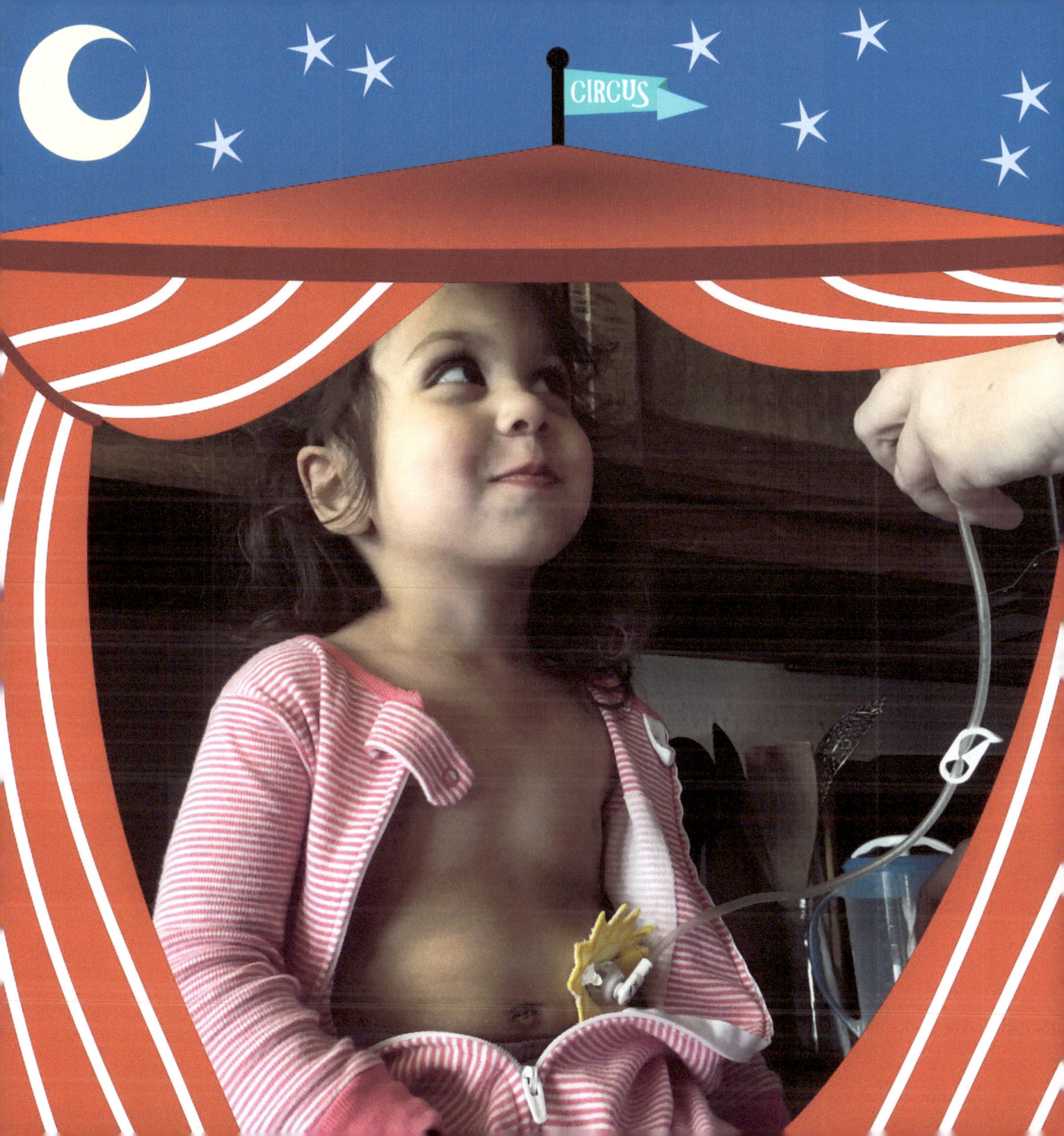

The flag reads: CIRCUS

Now that I'm all powered up, I can't wait to see what I'll do next.

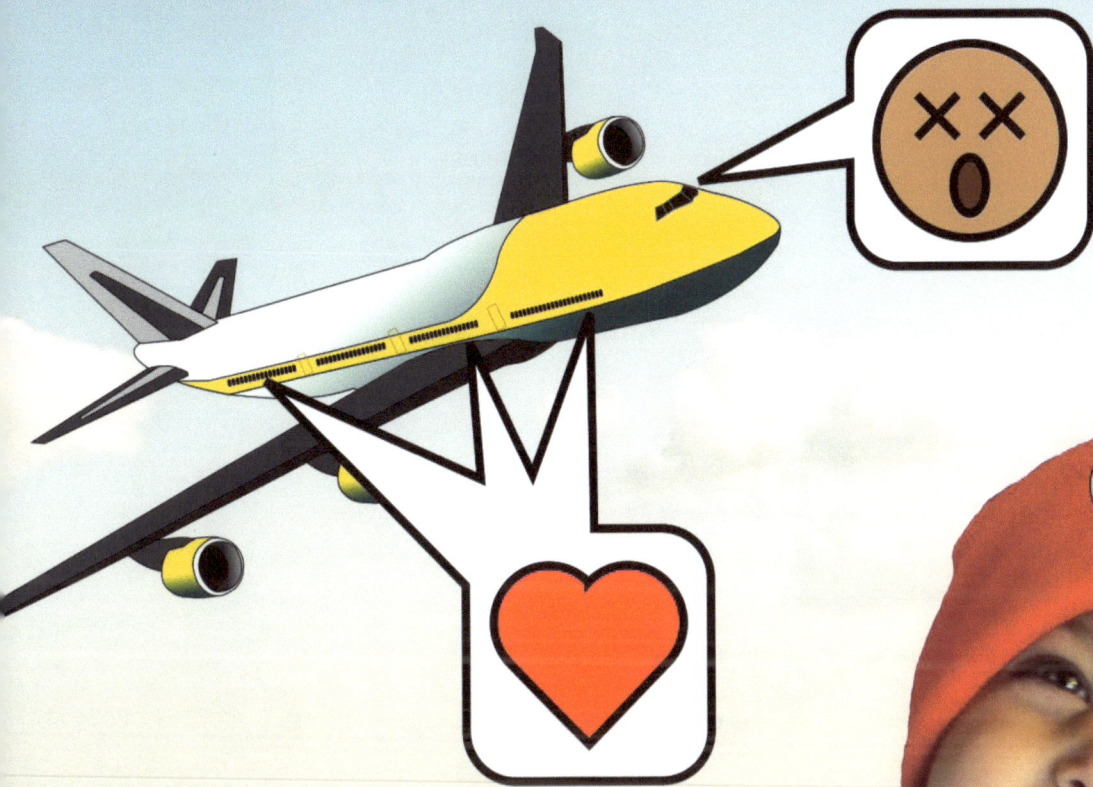

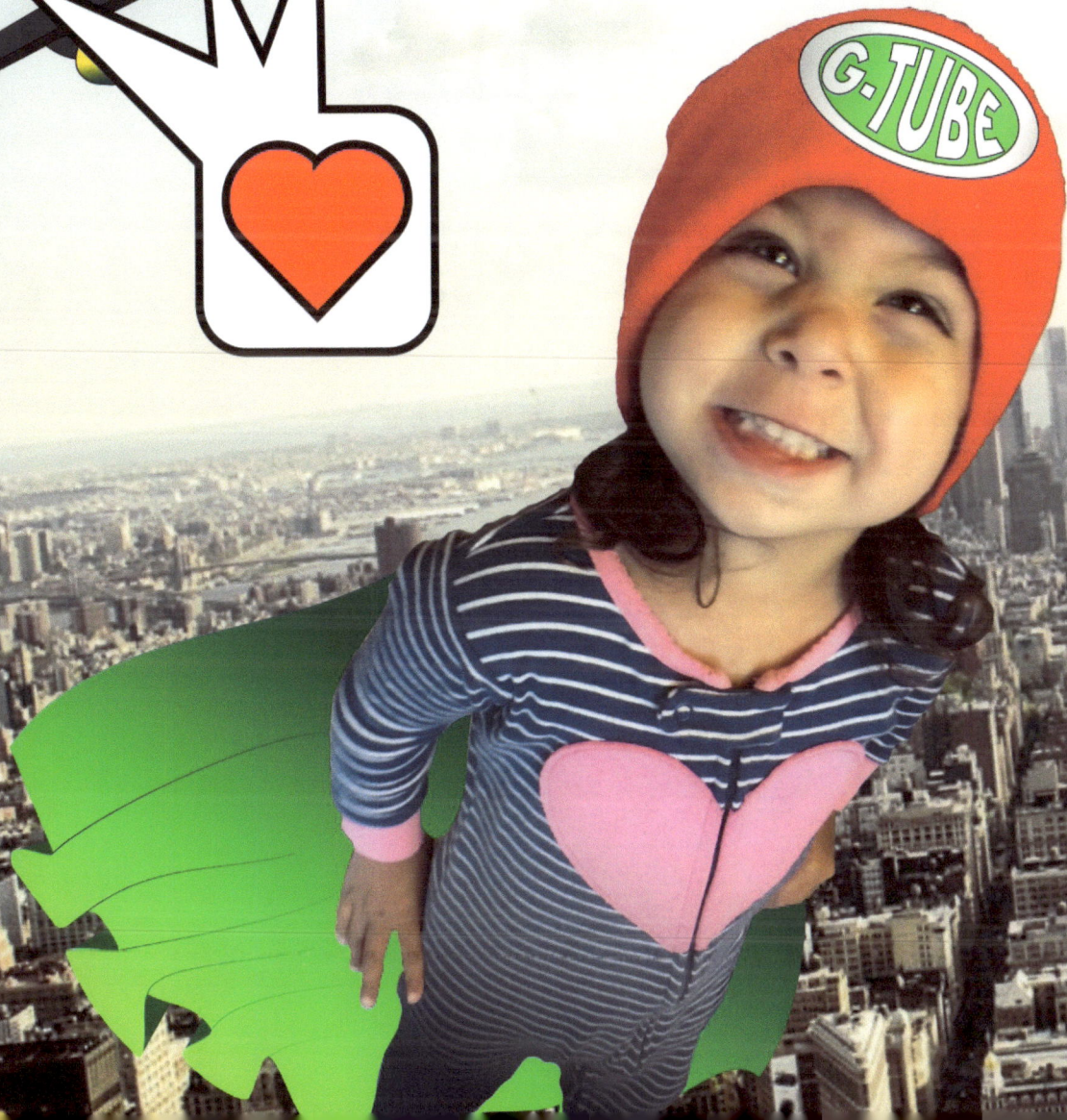

Gee whiz,
it'll be an
adventure.

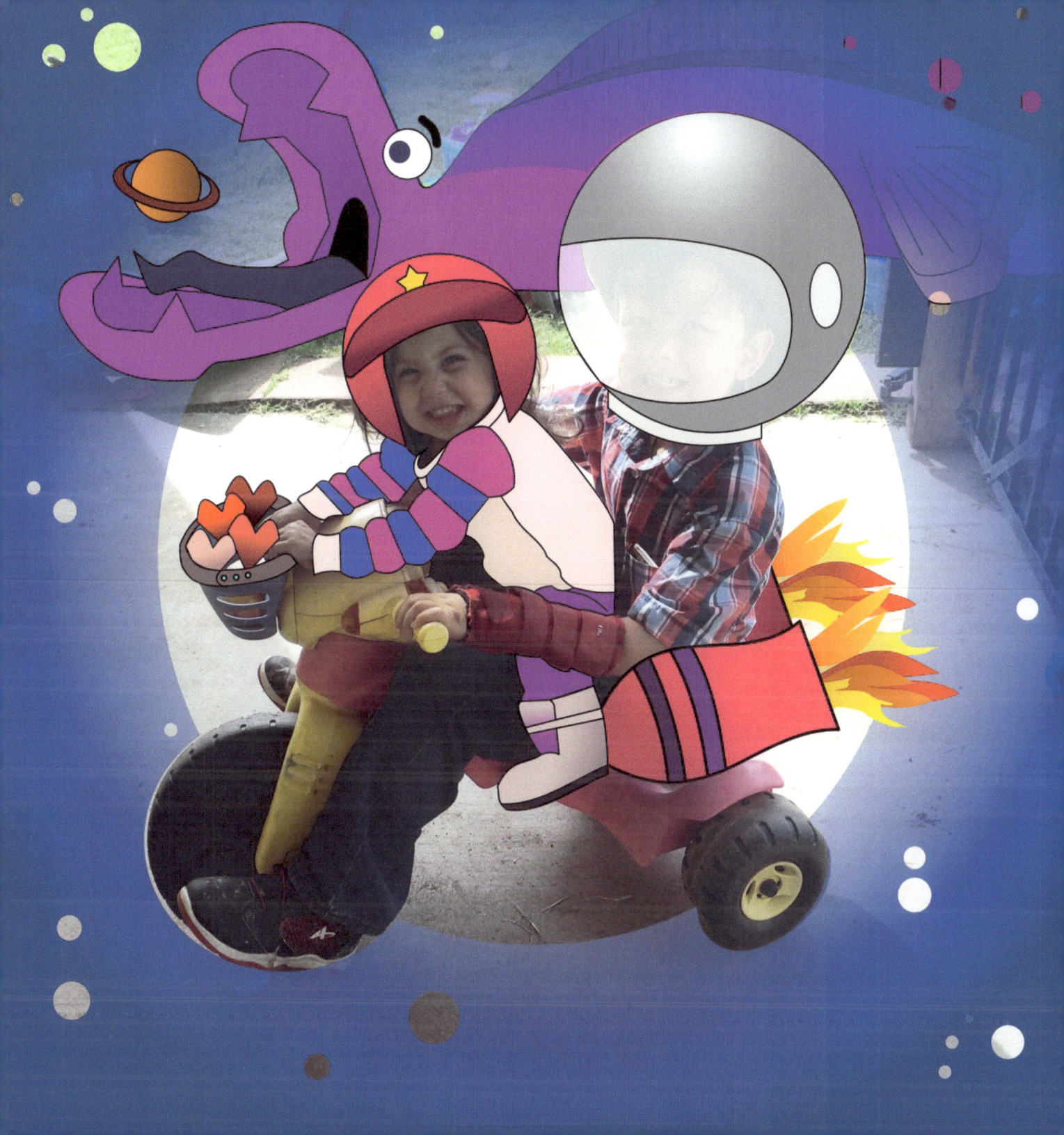

First Printing: 2017

ISBN: 978-0-9977588-8-7

HWC Press, LLC
P.O. Box 3792
Bartlesville, OK 74006

housewifeclass@gmail.com
www.housewifeclass.com
@housewifeclass

Ordering Information:

U.S. trade bookstores and wholesalers, please contact HWC Press. Special discounts are available on quantity purchase by corporations, association, educators, and others.

About the typefaces:

KOMIKA TITLE – PAINT, by Apostrophic Lab (https://www.ffonts.net/Komika-Title-Paint.font)

Minya Nouvelle, by Raymond Larabie (http://typodermicfonts.com/nouvelle-minya-nouvelle/)

BLOWBRUSH, by Petar Acanski (https://www.behance.net/gallery/33043073/BlowBrush-free-font)

DIGITAL DREAM, by Pizzadude (http://www.1001fonts.com/digital-dream-font.html)

HELLO DENVER, by Good Apples (http://www.1001fonts.com/hello-denver-display-font.html)

Crafty Girls, by Tart Workshop (http://www.1001fonts.com/crafty-girls-font.html)

AR Christy, by Arphic Technology (https://www.azfonts.net/load_font/ar-christy.html)